The Mayo Clinic Diet Blueprint

Tasty recipes and strategies for healthy living to reshape your life, with science-based habits while eating well, enjoying life and also losing weight.

Donna Johnson

Copyright 2023-

Donna Johnson

ISBN

Printed in the United States of America

Disclaimer

This publication is designed to provide competent and reliable information regarding the subject covered However, the views expressed in this publication are those of the author alone and should not be taken as expert instruction or professional advice The reader is responsible for his or her actions The author hereby disclaims any responsibility or liability whatsoever that is incurred from the use or application of the contents of this publication by the purchaser of the reader. The purchaser or reader is hereby responsible for his or her actions.

All rights reserved. No part of this publication may be reproduced, distributed or transmitted in any form or by any means, including photocopying, recording or other electronic or mechanical methods without the prior written permission of the publisher except in the case of owner quotations embodied in critical reviews and certain other non-commercial uses permitted by copyright law For permission requests write to the publisher addressed at the address below

Table of Contents

INTRODUCTION

Health is the weave and weight is the weft of the large tapestry that is our life; the careful balance between both dictates the quality of our trip. Your search for this book, "The Mayo Clinic Diet Blueprint: Your Weight Loss Journey," demonstrates a deep dedication to changing your story and taking back your vitality in addition to your goal to lose weight. We ask you to set out on a journey that goes beyond the numbers on a scale as you approach this life-changing experience. It's a route that will get you closer to a more vibrant, joyful, and healthy version of yourself.

There is no diet like the Mayo Clinic Diet that you have ever seen. It's not a passing trend, nor does it promise miraculous, instantaneous change. Rather, it is a methodically designed road map, an all-inclusive manual, and a reliable ally for your extraordinary weight loss expedition.

Setting out on a weight reduction quest means stepping into unfamiliar territory and a world full of deceptive trends and marketing. It's a place where you might feel lost and confused, with irritation and uncertainty often overshadowing progress. But you will also find the firm hand of science, the counsel of professionals, and the encouragement of a community committed to your achievement inside the pages of this book.

The foundation of "The Mayo Clinic Diet Blueprint" is the ageless idea of evidence-based nutrition and healthy living. It provides you with more than just a diet plan; it gives you a revolutionary approach to wellbeing that aims to create lifelong habits. This is a journey that goes beyond the scope of quick fixes, with the ultimate aims of transforming your relationship with food, motivating long-term lifestyle adjustments, and giving you the ability to take charge of your health.

This book is not meant to reassure you that it is simple. Sustainable weight reduction is a difficult journey that calls for perseverance, commitment, and a readiness to learn. However, the road has equal rewards in store, like increased self-assurance, an endless supply of energy, and the possibility of writing your own health narrative in the future.

Discover the mysteries of the Mayo Clinic Diet, which has changed the lives of many people, as you read through these pages. We'll explore the science behind its efficacy, get you ready for the special diet stages, and lead you through mouthwatering meal plans and dishes that will fuel your trip while tantalizing your taste buds.

But this is a guide for personal development, not simply a cookbook. It serves as a reminder that your health is your most valuable possession and that investing in it now will pay you in the long run. It's an honoring of the amazing potential that lies inside you and is just waiting to be realized.

Your path is as distinct as you are. The Mayo Clinic Diet Blueprint is flexible enough to accommodate your requirements, tastes, and schedule. It's a journey that gives you a feeling of agency and a renewed understanding of the need of self-care in addition to physical development.

As we go, you will come across motivational accounts of people who have traversed this route and come out on the other side, transformed both physically and spiritually. Their stories serve as a reminder of the opportunities that lie ahead.

Are you prepared to go above the norm and take control of your weight reduction journey? Are you ready to change the course of your life and take little steps toward rediscovering your vitality? If so, turn over a new leaf and embark on a significant journey with "The Mayo Clinic Diet Blueprint" as your guide. Awaiting you is your journey.

Part I:

Getting Started

Chapter 1
Setting the Stage for Success

Defining Your Weight Loss Goals

Establishing your weight reduction objectives is similar to drawing a route on a map before starting a trip. It's about outlining not only your destination but also your plan for getting there and the experiences you want to have along the way. It is essential that you approach this assignment with a combination of ambition, practicality, and a thorough awareness of your own goals.

1. Clarity and Specificity: Clearly defined objectives are essential. Rather of saying "I want to lose weight," try saying something more precise, like "I aim to lose 20 pounds in six months." As a beacon, clarity directs your efforts and keeps you on task.

2. Realistic Expectations: Although having desire is wonderful, your objectives have to be based on facts. Establish healthy and attainable goals. Setting unrealistic expectations might cause disappointment and cause your efforts to fail.

3. Take Into Account Non-Scale Objectives: Losing weight is about more than just the numbers on a scale. Think of additional success markers, such more vitality, better-fitting clothes, or general health gains. These non-scale successes are just as significant

and may serve as inspiration in ways that go beyond weight measurements.

4. Long-Term Vision: Establish both immediate and long-term objectives. While long-term objectives provide a vision for ongoing health and well-being, short-term goals keep you motivated and give you milestones to celebrate.

5. Health-Centric Approach: Give your health priority above looks. Rather of focusing just on getting to a specific dress size or weight on the scale, think about setting objectives that will help you feel better, have more energy, and lower your chance of health problems.

6. Behavioral Objectives: Think about the habits and behaviors required to reach your objectives in addition to the final product. Setting objectives like eating more veggies or exercising three times a week puts more emphasis on doable actions than just the final result.

7. Adaptability and Review: Be flexible with your objectives. Your attitude to objectives should be dynamic, just like life itself. Review and revise your objectives often to reflect evolving situations or fresh realizations encountered along the way.

Recall that your weight reduction experience is distinct and personal. You may not benefit from what works for someone else. As a result, give yourself enough time to reflect, comprehend your driving forces, and create objectives that really fit your desires and way of life. You're not only choosing a destination when you carefully consider and analyze your weight reduction objectives; you're also laying out a route that will lead to a better, happier, and more confident version of yourself.

Starting a weight reduction journey may be a difficult undertaking full with difficulties and roadblocks that can discourage even the most motivated people. However, having long-term success requires comprehending and knowing how to get beyond these typical obstacles to weight reduction. It's similar to negotiating a dangerous mountainous terrain, where being aware of possible hazards and equipped to avoid them might be crucial. Here, we examine these obstacles and provide special advice on how to overcome them:

1. Frustration and Plateaus: Plagues in weight loss refer to the dips in your trip when it looks like the scale is stuck and you don't make any progress. To get through this, keep in mind that plateaus are normal and often indicate that your body is changing. To spice things up, be patient, concentrate on non-scale successes, and think about changing your diet or exercise regimen.
2. Emotional Eating: Stress, melancholy, or even happiness may set off emotional eating,

which can be a formidable foe. Become emotionally aware in order to overcome this, and look for other coping strategies such as physical activity, meditation, or chatting to a friend. You may find trends by keeping a food diary.

3. Social Pressures and Peer Influence: Maintaining your weight reduction objectives might be difficult while dealing with social events, peer pressure, and cultural standards. Share your goals with loved ones, enlist their help, and make bold decisions that are healthy.

4. Time Constraints: Exercise and food preparation are often neglected due to hectic schedules. By putting your health first, making time for exercises like appointments, and using time-saving techniques like food preparation, you can get beyond this obstacle.

5. Lack of Motivation: It might be difficult to stay motivated while trying to lose weight. To get over this, make short-term objectives, give yourself praise when you succeed, and keep in mind why you set out on this adventure in the first place. Positive self-talk and visualization techniques may help increase motivation.

6. Cravings and Temptation: Although food cravings might be strong, you can manage them by recognizing your triggers, choosing

healthier alternatives in place of harmful ones, and engaging in mindful eating.

7. Lack of responsibility: In the absence of responsibility, it's simple to veer off course. Join a support group, find an accountability partner, or think about getting expert assistance from a personal trainer or nutritionist.

8. Injuries and Health Issues: Injury or pre-existing medical issues may prevent you from moving on. Consult a medical expert for advice on safe and efficient ways to adjust your weight reduction regimen.

9. Overly Restrictive Diets: Excessively restrictive diets might cause failure and exhaustion. Become over this obstacle by embracing a sustainable, well-balanced diet. For instance, the Mayo Clinic Diet promotes a balanced, pleasurable, and simpler diet to follow.

10. Negative Self-Talk and Self-Doubt: These two things may be quite crippling. Develop your sense of self-worth, self-acceptance, and self-compassion. Be in a positive environment and, if necessary, seek expert assistance.

Chapter 2

The Science behind the Mayo Clinic Diet

How the Diet Works

The Mayo Clinic Diet is a well-known and well-respected method to weight loss and general wellness. It is founded on the concepts of healthy eating, portion management, and progressive, long-term weight reduction. The Mayo Clinic Diet works as follows:

1. The Mayo Clinic Philosophy: Although not affiliated with the Mayo Clinic medical institution, the Mayo Clinic Diet is based on the clinic's healthy living philosophy. It highlights that reducing weight and sustaining a healthy lifestyle need more than simply eating less; it also requires making long-term, sustainable adjustments to your eating habits and daily routines.

2. Two-Phase Strategy:

   - Phase 1: Let It Go! This first phase is intended to kick-start your weight reduction. It's a two-week period during which you should drop 6 to 10 pounds. It focuses on breaking bad eating habits and replacing them with good ones. During this stage, you are urged to incorporate good habits into your daily routine, such as eating breakfast every day, exercising, and establishing attainable objectives. It includes meal planning and recipes to get you started.

- Phase 2: Experience It! Following the first phase, you go on to the "Live It!" phase, which is intended for long-term weight control. This phase does not have a time restriction since it reflects a long-term manner of eating. It promotes a wider range of foods and supports balanced, portion-controlled meals. The focus is on eating healthily, enjoying your meals, and leading an active lifestyle.

3. Food Options: The Mayo Clinic Diet emphasizes genuine, healthy foods found in your local grocery store. It promotes eating fruits and vegetables, entire grains, lean meats, and healthy fats. Because the diet does not depend on pre-packaged foods or supplements, it is a practical and cost-effective approach to healthy eating.

4. No Calorie Counting: This diet does not need calorie counting. It instead encourages portion management and attentive eating. You naturally minimize your calorie consumption by concentrating on the sorts of meals you consume and establishing better eating habits.

5. Daily Physical exercise: The Mayo Clinic Diet encourages physical exercise as an important component of living a healthy lifestyle. It suggests 30 minutes of moderate exercise every day. Exercise is important not

just for weight reduction, but also for general health and well-being.

6. Support and Community: The Mayo Clinic Diet gives you access to a helpful online community as well as resources. You may connect with others on the same road, exchange stories, find encouragement, and get professional advice.

7. Individualization: Because everyone is different, the diet may be tailored to individual tastes, dietary limitations, and health requirements. Because of its adaptability, it is accessible to a broad spectrum of individuals.

8. Scientific Foundation: Although not affiliated with the Mayo Clinic, the diet is founded on scientific principles and encourages evidence-based nutrition and health practices.

Benefits of the Diet

The Mayo Clinic Diet has various advantages for those who want to lose weight and keep it off, as well as enhance their general health. The following are some of the main advantages of the Mayo Clinic Diet:

1. Sustainable Weight reduction: The Mayo Clinic Diet is intended to promote progressive, long-term weight reduction. It focuses on long-term adjustments to your food and activity habits, lowering your chance

of regaining weight, which is typical with many fad diets.

2. Healthy Eating Habits: The diet emphasizes entire foods such as fruits, vegetables, whole grains, lean meats, and healthy fats. This promotes a well-balanced, healthy diet.
3. No Calorie Counting: The Mayo Clinic Diet does not need calorie counting. It promotes portion management and mindful eating instead, making it a more realistic and achievable strategy for many people.
4. Emphasis on Physical exercise: The diet emphasizes frequent physical exercise, which aids in not just weight loss but also fitness and general health.
5. No pricey Supplements or Foods: The Mayo Clinic Diet does not depend on pricey, specialty foods or supplements. It is based on genuine, daily items that can be found at your local grocery store, making it both affordable and accessible.
6. Good Lifestyle Changes: The diet supports the adoption of good lifestyle changes such as eating breakfast, establishing reasonable objectives, and enjoying your meals, in addition to what you consume.
7. Flexible and Adaptable: Because the Mayo Clinic Diet is adaptable to individual tastes, dietary limitations, and health concerns, it is suitable for a broad spectrum of individuals.

8. Evidence-founded Approach: Although not affiliated with the Mayo Clinic, the diet is founded on scientific principles and encourages evidence-based nutrition and health practices.

9. Improved Overall Health: The Mayo Clinic Diet may lead to improved overall health by concentrating on a balanced diet and frequent physical exercise. This includes better cardiovascular health, lower blood pressure, and a decreased risk of chronic illnesses.

10. Better Nutritional Understanding: The diet teaches you about nutrition and assists you in making educated food choices, allowing you to sustain a healthy lifestyle outside of the diet program.

11. Personalization: Because each person's demands and tastes are unique, the diet allows you to personalize the program to your own lifestyle.

Chapter 3
Preparing Your Mind and Kitchen

Mental Preparation

Starting the Mayo Clinic Diet is more than just a physical journey; it's also a fundamental adjustment in perspective and a commitment to supporting your mental well-being. You must be psychologically prepared to succeed in this attempt. Here's a thorough and one-of-a-kind description of how to psychologically prepare for the Mayo Clinic Diet:

1. Explain Your "Why": Take some time to consider your motives before beginning the Mayo Clinic Diet. Why do you wish to go on this adventure? When difficulties emerge, your "why" serves as an anchor and source of drive. It might be to enhance your health, raise your confidence, or set a good example for your family. Understanding your "why" will assist you in remaining committed.

2. Create reasonable Expectations: Part of mental preparation is creating reasonable expectations. Understand that the Mayo Clinic Diet is not a fast cure; rather, it is a steady and long-term strategy to weight loss. Accept that there will be ups and downs, and that meaningful changes may take time.

3. Mindful Goal Setting: Rather than concentrating entirely on the final goal, establish smaller, more manageable goals. Divide your trip into doable chunks.

Celebrating tiny triumphs will give you a feeling of achievement and desire to keep going.

4. Positive Self-Talk: Be mindful of your inner dialogue. Self-doubt and negative self-talk can be major barriers to success. Practice positive affirmations and cultivate self-compassion. Instead of berating yourself for slip-ups, acknowledge them as learning opportunities.

5. Visualize Success: Use the power of visualization to see yourself succeeding on the Mayo Clinic Diet. Envision a healthier, happier version of yourself, and picture the positive impact on your life. This mental exercise can boost motivation and reinforce your commitment.

6. Mental Resilience: Weight loss journeys are not without challenges. Develop mental resilience to overcome setbacks. Understand that occasional slip-ups are normal, and they don't define your journey. Learn from them and keep moving forward.

7. Social Support: Share your goals with friends and family, and seek their support. Having a network of people who understand and encourage your journey can provide valuable emotional reinforcement.

8. Coping Strategies: Identify healthy coping strategies for managing stress or emotional triggers without resorting to emotional eating.

Consider activities like meditation, yoga, or talking to a therapist if needed.

9. Education and Preparation: Educate yourself about the Mayo Clinic Diet, including the science behind it and the practical aspects of the program. Knowledge empowers you to make informed choices and reduces anxiety.
10. Flexibility and Adaptability: Understand that not every day will go as planned. Be flexible and adaptable to unforeseen circumstances. Don't let one setback derail your progress. Instead, find creative solutions to stay on track.
11. Self-Care: Prioritize self-care. Weight loss can be demanding, both physically and mentally. Ensure you're getting enough rest, relaxation, and moments of self-indulgence to recharge and stay motivated.
12. Accountability and Tracking: Consider maintaining a journal or using a mobile app to track your progress. Keeping a record of your meals, exercise, and emotions can help you stay accountable and identify patterns in your behavior.

Stocking Your Pantry and Fridge

Stocking your pantry and refrigerator for the Mayo Clinic Diet is an important step in ensuring that you have the necessary supplies on hand to prepare nutritious and tasty meals. Here's a thorough guide to equipping your kitchen for Mayo Clinic Diet success:

Pantry Essentials:

1.	Whole Grains:	- Brown rice - Quinoa - Whole wheat pasta - Oats - Whole grain cereals
2	Canned or Dried Legumes:	- Lentils - Chickpeas - Black beans - Kidney beans
3	Healthy Oils:	- Extra virgin olive oil - Canola oil - Coconut oil (for occasional use)
4	Herbs and Spices:	An assortment of herbs and spices like basil, oregano, thyme, cumin, paprika, and more for flavoring dishes without excess salt or sugar.
5	Low-Sodium Broths:	- Vegetable broth - Chicken or turkey broth (if not following a vegetarian diet)
6	Nuts and Seeds:	- Almonds, walnuts, chia seeds, flaxseeds

		- Nut butters without added sugars or salt
7	Canned Tomatoes and Tomato Sauce:	- Choose options without added sugars and salt.
8	Whole-Grain Flour:	- Whole wheat flour or alternative flours like almond or coconut for baking
9	Vinegars:	- Balsamic, red wine, and apple cider vinegar for dressings and marinades.

Refrigerator Essentials:

1	Fresh Produce	- A variety of vegetables such as leafy greens, tomatoes, cucumbers, bell peppers, carrots, and broccoli. - Fresh fruits like berries, apples, citrus fruits, and bananas.
2	Lean Proteins:	- Skinless poultry (chicken or turkey) - Lean cuts of beef or pork (in moderation) - Fish (salmon, tilapia, or other varieties)

		- Eggs - Low-fat or Greek yogurt
3	Low-Fat Dairy:	- Low-fat milk or dairy alternatives like almond or soy milk
4	Tofu or Tempeh:	- For vegetarian sources of protein
5	Fresh Herbs:	- Stock up on fresh herbs like basil, cilantro, and parsley to add flavor to dishes.
6	Condiments:	- Mustard, low-sodium soy sauce, and hot sauce (in moderation)

Freezer Essentials:

1.	Frozen Vegetables	- Frozen broccoli, spinach, peas, and mixed vegetable blends are convenient options.
2.	Lean Proteins:	- Store extra portions of lean proteins in the freezer for easy meal planning.
3.	Berries:	- Frozen berries for smoothies or oatmeal.

4.	Whole Wheat Bread:	- Store extra loaves of whole wheat bread in the freezer to keep them fresh.

Additional Tips:

1. Check Labels: When shopping, check food labels carefully to verify that you're selecting goods with no added sugars, little salt, and few processed ingredients.
2. Meal Planning: Plan your meals ahead of time and create a shopping list to minimize impulsive purchases and ensure you have all the components.
3. Portion management: Purchase measuring cups and a kitchen scale to aid with portion management and to verify you're adhering to the Mayo Clinic Diet recommendations.

Part II:

Recipes and Meal Plans

Chapter 4
Delicious and Nutritious Breakfasts

Recipe 1. Greek Yogurt Parfait:

Ingredients:

- Low-fat Greek yogurt
- Fresh berries (e.g., strawberries, blueberries)
- Honey or a drizzle of pure maple syrup
- Chopped nuts (e.g., almonds or walnuts)

Instructions:

1. In a glass or bowl, layer Greek yogurt, fresh berries, and a drizzle of honey or maple syrup.
2. Top with chopped nuts for added crunch and flavor.

Preparation time is about 5 minutes

Recipe 2. Oatmeal with Apples and Cinnamon:

Ingredients:

- Rolled oats
- Sliced apples
- Ground cinnamon
- Chopped nuts (e.g., walnuts or almonds)

Instructions:

1. Cook rolled oats with water or low-fat milk.
2. Top with sliced apples, a sprinkle of ground cinnamon, and a handful of chopped nuts.

Preparation time is about 25 to 30 minutes

Recipe 3. Whole Wheat Pancakes:

Ingredients:

- Whole wheat flour
- Baking powder
- Low-fat milk or dairy alternative
- Egg or egg substitute
- Vanilla extract

Instructions:

1. Mix whole wheat flour, baking powder, low-fat milk, an egg (or egg substitute), and a dash of vanilla extract to make pancake batter.
2. Cook on a non-stick griddle or pan.
3. Top with fresh berries and a dollop of Greek yogurt.

Preparation time is about 30 minutes

Recipe 4. Vegetable Omelet:

Ingredients:

- Eggs or egg whites
- Chopped vegetables (e.g., bell peppers, spinach, tomatoes)
- Onion
- Low-fat cheese (optional)

Instructions:

1. Whisk eggs or egg whites and pour them into a hot, non-stick skillet.
2. Add chopped vegetables and cook until set.
3. Optionally, add a sprinkle of low-fat cheese before folding the omelet in half.

Preparation time is about 10 to 15 minutes

Recipe 5. Chia Seed Pudding:

Ingredients:

- Chia seeds
- Low-fat milk or almond milk
- Vanilla extract
- Fresh fruit (e.g., sliced bananas or mixed berries)

Instructions:

1. Mix chia seeds with milk and a dash of vanilla extract in a jar or bowl.
2. Refrigerate overnight until it thickens.
3. Top with fresh fruit before serving.

Preparation time is about 5 minutes

Recipe 6. Whole Wheat Toast with Avocado and Poached Egg:

Ingredients:

- Whole wheat toast
- Ripe avocado
- Poached egg

- Salt and pepper

Instructions:

1. Mash ripe avocado and spread it on whole wheat toast.
2. Top with a perfectly poached egg and season with salt and pepper.

Preparation time is about 10 minutes

Recipe 7. Green Smoothie:

Ingredients:

- Spinach or kale
- Banana
- Low-fat yogurt
- Honey (optional)
- Ice cubes

Instructions:

1. Blend spinach or kale, a ripe banana, low-fat yogurt, honey (if desired), and ice cubes until smooth.

Preparation time is about 5 minutes

Chapter 5

Energizing Lunches and Snacks

Energizing Lunch Recipes

Recipe 8. Mediterranean Chickpea Salad:

Ingredients:

- Canned chickpeas (rinsed and drained)
- Chopped cucumbers
- Cherry tomatoes, halved
- Kalamata olives, pitted and sliced
- Red onion, thinly sliced
- Fresh parsley, chopped
- Feta cheese, crumbled (optional)
- Lemon vinaigrette (made with lemon juice, olive oil, salt, and pepper)

Instructions:

1. In a large bowl, combine chickpeas, cucumbers, cherry tomatoes, Kalamata olives, red onion, and fresh parsley.
2. Drizzle with the lemon vinaigrette and toss to coat. If desired, top with crumbled feta cheese.

Preparation time is about 10 to 15 minutes

Recipe 9. Turkey and Avocado Wrap:

Ingredients:

- Sliced turkey breast
- Sliced avocado

- Whole wheat tortilla or lettuce leaves (for a low-carb option)
- Sliced tomatoes
- Lettuce or spinach
- Greek yogurt or mustard for spread

Instructions:

1. Lay out the tortilla or lettuce leaf and spread with Greek yogurt or mustard.
2. Place sliced turkey, avocado, sliced tomatoes, and lettuce or spinach.
3. Roll it up and slice for a protein-rich and satisfying lunch.

Preparation time is about 10 minutes

Recipe 10. Quinoa and Vegetable Stir-Fry:

Ingredients:

- Cooked quinoa
- Sliced bell peppers (various colors)
- Broccoli florets
- Carrot strips
- Snow peas
- Low-sodium soy sauce
- Ginger and garlic for flavor

Instructions:

1. In a hot pan, stir-fry the sliced bell peppers, broccoli, carrot strips, and snow peas with a

splash of low-sodium soy sauce, ginger, and garlic.
2. Serve over cooked quinoa for a nutritious and filling lunch.

Preparation time is about 30 to 40 minutes

Recipe 11. Spinach and Strawberry Salad:

Ingredients:

- Baby spinach leaves
- Sliced strawberries
- Sliced almonds
- Red onion, thinly sliced
- Feta cheese, crumbled (optional)
- Balsamic vinaigrette dressing

Instructions:

1. In a large bowl, combine baby spinach, sliced strawberries, sliced almonds, red onion, and crumbled feta cheese.
2. Drizzle with balsamic vinaigrette dressing for a fresh and vibrant salad.

Preparation time is about 15 to 20 minutes

Recipe 12. Tuna and White Bean Salad:

Ingredients:

- Canned tuna in water, drained
- Canned white beans (cannellini or Great Northern), rinsed and drained

- Chopped celery
- Chopped red onion
- Lemon juice
- Olive oil
- Fresh parsley, chopped
- Salt and pepper

Instructions:

1. In a bowl, combine tuna, white beans, chopped celery, chopped red onion, and fresh parsley.
2. Drizzle with lemon juice and olive oil. Season with salt and pepper.

Preparation time is about 15 to 20 minutes

Recipe 13. Grilled Vegetable and Quinoa Bowl:

Ingredients:

- Grilled vegetables (zucchini, eggplant, bell peppers)
- Cooked quinoa
- Fresh basil or mint leaves
- Balsamic glaze or dressing

Instructions:

1. Arrange grilled vegetables and quinoa in a bowl.
2. Top with fresh basil or mint leaves and drizzle with balsamic glaze or dressing.

Preparation time is about 30 to 40 minutes

Recipe 14. Smoked Salmon and Cucumber Roll-Ups:

Ingredients:

- Smoked salmon slices
- Cucumber slices
- Low-fat cream cheese (optional)
- Fresh dill (optional)

Instructions:

1. Lay out a smoked salmon slice and place a cucumber slice on top.
2. Optionally, spread with low-fat cream cheese and sprinkle with fresh dill.
3. Roll it up for a light and protein-packed lunch.

Preparation time is about 15 to 20 minutes

Recipe 15. Quinoa and Chickpea Salad:

Ingredients:

- Cooked quinoa
- Chickpeas
- Chopped cucumbers
- Cherry tomatoes
- Red onion, finely diced
- Fresh parsley, chopped
- Lemon vinaigrette (made with lemon juice, olive oil, salt, and pepper)

Instructions:

1. In a large bowl, combine quinoa, chickpeas, cucumbers, cherry tomatoes, red onion, and fresh parsley.
2. Drizzle with the lemon vinaigrette and toss to coat. Adjust seasoning to taste.

Preparation time is about 25 to 40 minutes

Recipe 16. Grilled Chicken and Vegetable Wrap:

Ingredients:

- Grilled chicken breast strips
- Whole wheat tortilla or lettuce leaves (for a low-carb option)
- Sliced tomatoes
- Lettuce or spinach
- Cucumber, sliced
- Greek yogurt or hummus for spread

Instructions:

1. Lay out the tortilla or lettuce leaf and spread with Greek yogurt or hummus.
2. Place grilled chicken strips, sliced tomatoes, lettuce or spinach, and sliced cucumber.
3. Wrap it up and slice for a convenient and protein-packed lunch.

Preparation time is about 20 to 30 minutes

Recipe 17. Black Bean and Corn Salad:

Ingredients:

- Canned black beans (rinsed and drained)
- Corn kernels (fresh or thawed if frozen)
- Diced red onions
- Chopped cilantro
- Lime juice and a dash of olive oil

Instructions:

1. Mix black beans, corn, diced onions, and cilantro in a bowl.
2. Drizzle with lime juice and a dash of olive oil for a zesty salad.

Preparation time is about 10 to 15 minutes

Recipe 18. Mediterranean Quinoa Bowl:

Ingredients:

- Cooked quinoa
- Sliced cucumbers
- Cherry tomatoes, halved
- Kalamata olives, pitted
- Feta cheese, crumbled
- Red onion, thinly sliced
- Fresh basil or mint leaves
- Lemon juice and olive oil for dressing

Instructions:

1. In a bowl, combine quinoa, cucumbers, cherry tomatoes, Kalamata olives, crumbled feta cheese, red onion, and fresh basil or mint leaves.

2. Drizzle with lemon juice and olive oil, and toss to combine.

Preparation time is about 25 to 30 minutes

Recipe 19. Tuna Salad Lettuce Wraps:

Ingredients:

- Canned tuna in water, drained
- Greek yogurt (or light mayonnaise)
- Diced celery
- Diced red onion
- Pickles, diced
- Lettuce leaves (such as Romaine or iceberg)

Instructions:

1. In a bowl, mix the tuna, Greek yogurt (or light mayonnaise), diced celery, diced red onion, and pickles.
2. Spoon the tuna salad into lettuce leaves and roll them up for a low-carb and protein-rich lunch.

Preparation time is about 10 to 15 minutes

Energizing Snacks Recipes

Recipe 20. Cottage Cheese and Pineapple:

Ingredients:

- Low-fat cottage cheese
- Chunks of fresh pineapple

Instructions:

1. Enjoy a serving of low-fat cottage cheese with chunks of fresh pineapple for a sweet and savory snack.

Preparation time is about 5 to 10 minutes

Recipe 21. Greek Yogurt with Berries:

Ingredients:

- Low-fat Greek yogurt
- Fresh berries (strawberries, blueberries, raspberries)
- Optional: a drizzle of honey or a sprinkle of nuts

Instructions:

1. Top low-fat Greek yogurt with a generous portion of fresh berries for a protein-packed and nutritious snack.
2. If desired, add a drizzle of honey or a sprinkle of nuts for extra flavor.

Preparation time is about 5 to 10 minutes

Recipe 22. Hummus and Vegetable Sticks:

Ingredients:

- Carrot sticks
- Cucumber sticks
- Bell pepper strips
- Cherry tomatoes
- Snap peas

- Hummus for dipping

Instructions:

1. Serve an assortment of vegetable sticks and cherry tomatoes with a side of hummus for a crunchy and satisfying snack.

Preparation time is about 15 to 20 minutes, depending on whether you make the hummus from scratch or use store-bought hummus.

Recipe 23. Mixed Nuts and Dried Fruits:

Ingredients:

- A mix of unsalted nuts (almonds, walnuts, pistachios)
- Dried fruits (apricots, cranberries, raisins)

Instructions:

1. Create a satisfying snack mix by combining a variety of unsalted nuts with dried fruits.
2. Portion it into small snack-sized containers for convenience.

Preparation time is about 5 to 10 minutes

Recipe 24. Smoothie Bowl:

Ingredients:

- Greek yogurt
- Blended fruit (banana, berries, or your choice)

- Toppings (chia seeds, sliced almonds, fresh fruit)

Instructions:

1. In a bowl, layer Greek yogurt and blended fruit to create a smoothie base.
2. Top with chia seeds, sliced almonds, and fresh fruit for a filling and customizable snack.

Preparation time is about 5 to 10 minutes

Recipe 25. Dark Chocolate and Almonds:

Ingredients:

- Dark chocolate with a high cocoa content
- Raw or roasted almonds

Instructions:

1. Enjoy a small piece of dark chocolate with a handful of raw or roasted almonds for a satisfying and heart-healthy snack.

Preparation time is about 5 to 15 minutes

Recipe 26. Apple Slices with Almond Butter:

Ingredients:

- Apple slices
- Almond butter (or any nut or seed butter)

Instructions:

1. Dip apple slices in almond butter for a fiber-
    rich and energy-boosting snack.

Preparation time is about 5 to 15 minutes

Recipe 27. Grilled Lemon Herb Chicken:

Ingredients:

- Chicken breast or thighs
- Fresh lemon juice
- Olive oil
- Minced garlic
- Chopped fresh herbs (e.g., rosemary, thyme, parsley)
- Salt and pepper

Instructions:

1. In a bowl, combine lemon juice, olive oil, minced garlic, fresh herbs, salt, and pepper to create a marinade.
2. Marinate the chicken in the mixture for at least 30 minutes.
3. Grill the chicken until fully cooked. Serve with a side of steamed vegetables or a mixed greens salad.

Preparation time is about 20 to 25 minutes, depending on the thickness of the chicken pieces and the heat of your grill.

Recipe 28. Baked Salmon with Asparagus:

Ingredients:

- Salmon fillets

- Fresh asparagus spears
- Lemon slices
- Olive oil
- Dijon mustard
- Garlic powder
- Salt and pepper

Instructions:

1. Preheat the oven to 400°F (200°C).
2. In a bowl, whisk together olive oil, Dijon mustard, garlic powder, salt, and pepper.
3. Place salmon fillets on a baking sheet and arrange asparagus around them.
4. Brush the salmon and asparagus with the olive oil mixture, and top with lemon slices.
5. Bake for about 15-20 minutes or until the salmon flakes easily with a fork.

Preparation time is about 25 to 30 minutes, depending on the thickness of the salmon fillets and the desired level of doneness.

Recipe 29. Quinoa and Black Bean Stuffed Bell Peppers:

Ingredients:

- Bell peppers (various colors)
- Cooked quinoa
- Canned black beans (rinsed and drained)
- Diced tomatoes
- Salsa

- Ground cumin
- Chopped fresh cilantro
- Shredded low-fat cheese (optional)

Instructions:

1. Preheat the oven to 375°F (190°C).
2. Cut the tops off the bell peppers and remove the seeds.
3. In a bowl, mix cooked quinoa, black beans, diced tomatoes, salsa, ground cumin, and fresh cilantro.
4. Stuff the bell peppers with the quinoa and black bean mixture.
5. Optionally, top with shredded low-fat cheese.
6. Bake in a casserole dish for about 30-35 minutes or until the peppers are tender.

Preparation time is about 45 minutes to 1 hour, depending on the specific cooking times for the quinoa and the bell peppers.

Recipe 30. Vegetable Stir-Fry with Tofu:

Ingredients:

- Firm tofu, cubed
- Assorted vegetables (bell peppers, broccoli, snap peas, carrots)
- Low-sodium soy sauce
- Minced ginger and garlic
- Sesame oil
- Cooked brown rice or quinoa

Instructions:

1. In a wok or skillet, heat sesame oil and stir-fry tofu until golden brown. Remove from the pan.
2. Stir-fry a selection of vegetables with minced ginger and garlic until tender-crisp.
3. Add tofu back to the pan and drizzle with low-sodium soy sauce.
4. Serve the stir-fry over cooked brown rice or quinoa.

Preparation time is about 30 to 40 minutes

Recipe 31. Spaghetti Squash with Marinara Sauce:

Ingredients:

*   Spaghetti squash
*   Marinara sauce (choose one with no added sugars)
*   Grated Parmesan cheese (optional)
*   Fresh basil leaves

Instructions:

1. Cut the spaghetti squash in half, scoop out the seeds, and roast it in the oven until the flesh is tender.
2. Use a fork to scrape the squash into "noodles."
3. Heat marinara sauce and pour it over the spaghetti squash.

4. Optionally, sprinkle with grated Parmesan cheese and fresh basil.

Preparation time is about 1 hour 15 minutes, including the baking time for the spaghetti squash.

Recipe 32. Lean Beef and Vegetable Stir-Fry:

Ingredients:

- Lean beef strips
- Sliced bell peppers
- Sliced zucchini
- Sliced mushrooms
- Low-sodium stir-fry sauce
- Cooked brown rice or quinoa

Instructions:

1. Stir-fry lean beef in a hot skillet until cooked to your liking.
2. Add sliced bell peppers, zucchini, and mushrooms and stir-fry until tender.
3. Drizzle with low-sodium stir-fry sauce.
4. Serve over cooked brown rice or quinoa.

Preparation time is about 20 to 30 minutes, depending on the specific ingredients and the level of cooking you prefer.

Recipe 33. Baked Chicken with Roasted Vegetables:

Ingredients:

- Chicken thighs or breasts

- Assorted root vegetables (e.g., sweet potatoes, carrots, parsnips)
- Olive oil
- Dried rosemary and thyme
- Salt and pepper

Instructions:

1. Preheat the oven to 400°F (200°C).
2. Toss chicken and root vegetables in a mixture of olive oil, dried rosemary, dried thyme, salt, and pepper.
3. Arrange them on a baking sheet and bake until the chicken is cooked through and the vegetables are tender and caramelized.

Preparation time is about 45 minutes to 1 hour, depending on the size and thickness of the chicken pieces and the specific vegetables you are using.

Recipe 34. Berry Parfait:

Ingredients:

- Low-fat Greek yogurt
- Fresh mixed berries (e.g., strawberries, blueberries, raspberries)
- Honey or a drizzle of pure maple syrup

Instructions:

1. In a glass or bowl, layer low-fat Greek yogurt and fresh mixed berries.
2. Drizzle with honey or pure maple syrup for natural sweetness.

Preparation time is about 10 to 15 minutes

Recipe 35. Dark Chocolate-Dipped Strawberries:

Ingredients:

- Fresh strawberries
- Dark chocolate (70% cocoa or higher)
- Chopped nuts (e.g., almonds, pistachios)

Instructions:

1. Melt dark chocolate in a microwave or double boiler.
2. Dip fresh strawberries in the melted chocolate and roll them in chopped nuts.

3. Allow them to cool and harden before indulging.

Preparation time is about 15 to 20 minutes, but do allow additional time for the chocolate to set and harden.

Recipe 36. Chia Seed Pudding with Fresh Fruit:

Ingredients:

- Chia seeds
- Low-fat milk or almond milk
- Fresh fruit (e.g., sliced bananas, mixed berries)
- A drizzle of honey (optional)

Instructions:

1. Mix chia seeds with low-fat milk or almond milk and let it sit in the refrigerator until it thickens.
2. Top with fresh fruit and, if desired, a drizzle of honey.

Preparation time is about 10 to 30 minutes, plus freezing time of about 2 to 5 hours to thicken and develop a pudding like consistency.

Recipe 37. Baked Apples with Cinnamon:

Ingredients:

- Apples
- Ground cinnamon
- Chopped nuts (e.g., walnuts, pecans)

- A drizzle of honey (optional)

Instructions:

1. Preheat the oven to 375°F (190°C).
2. Core apples and sprinkle with ground cinnamon.
3. Fill the cores with chopped nuts and, optionally, a drizzle of honey.
4. Bake until the apples are soft and fragrant.

Preparation time is about 30 to 45 minutes

Recipe 38. Frozen Banana "Ice Cream":

Ingredients:

- Ripe bananas
- Optional add-ins: cocoa powder, peanut butter, vanilla extract

Instructions:

1. Slice ripe bananas and freeze until firm.
2. Blend the frozen banana slices until smooth.
3. Add optional add-ins like cocoa powder, peanut butter, or vanilla extract for flavor variations.

Preparation time is about 5 to 10 minutes, plus about 1 to 2 hours for freezing time.

Recipe 39. Greek Yogurt with Berries and a Drizzle of Agave:

Ingredients:

- Low-fat Greek yogurt
- Fresh berries (e.g., raspberries, blackberries)
- Agave nectar (or honey)

Instructions:

1. Top a serving of low-fat Greek yogurt with fresh berries.
2. Drizzle with agave nectar or honey for added sweetness.

Preparation time is about 10 to 30 minutes

Recipe 40. Pineapple Sorbet:

Ingredients:

- Fresh pineapple chunks
- Lime juice
- Fresh mint leaves

Instructions:

1. Blend fresh pineapple chunks with a splash of lime juice.
2. Freeze until it reaches a sorbet-like consistency.
3. Serve with fresh mint leaves for a refreshing dessert.

Preparation time is about 30 to 45 minutes, time required for freezing is about 2 to 4 hours.

Part III:

Staying on Track

Chapter 8

Strategies for Consistency

Consistency is key for long-term success while following the Mayo Clinic Diet, as it is with any healthy eating plan. Here are some tips to help you maintain consistency:

1. Establish Specific and Achievable Goals: Establish explicit, quantifiable, and attainable objectives. Having specific goals, whether it's decreasing weight or introducing more fruits and vegetables into your diet, can keep you motivated.

2. Develop a Meal Plan: Plan your meals ahead of time. When you're hungry and unprepared, this helps you make better meal choices and decreases the temptation to choose less nutritious alternatives.

3. Maintain a Healthy Kitchen: Stock your cupboard and refrigerator with items that adhere to the guidelines of the Mayo Clinic Diet. This makes it simpler to create nutritious meals and snacks.

4. Portion Management: Educate yourself on correct meal sizes and practice portion management. Using smaller dishes, weighing your meals, and paying attention to portion sizes may all help you control your calorie consumption.

5. Maintain a Food diary: Maintain a food diary to monitor your daily meals and snacks. This

may assist you in identifying trends, making improvements, and staying responsible.

6. Consistent eating Times: Maintain a regular eating plan. Eating at regular intervals may aid in the regulation of hunger and the prevention of overeating.
7. Stay Hydrated: Throughout the day, drink lots of water. Feelings of hunger may often be mistaken for indicators of dehydration.
8. Monitor Your Progress: Track your progress on a regular basis, whether via weigh-ins, measurements, or monitoring how your clothing fit. Along the journey, celebrate your accomplishments.
9. Discover Healthy Substitutes: Look for healthier alternatives to your favorite meals. with example, if you have a sweet craving, consider substituting naturally sweet fruits with sugary treats.
10. Include Variety: Include a wide range of foods in your diet. To keep your meals interesting and pleasurable, try out new recipes and components.
11. Social Support: Discuss your objectives with your friends and family. Having a support network might help you stick to your diet and remain motivated.
12. Stress Management: Stress may contribute to emotional eating. Find healthy stress-management methods, such as exercise, meditation, or relaxation techniques.

13. Plan for Special Occasions: Organize your approach to social events, parties, and special occasions. These events may be enjoyed without deviating from your diet.
14. Prepare nutritious Snacks: Keep nutritious snacks on hand for case hunger hits between meals. This keeps you from choosing harmful alternatives.
15. Be Patient and Kind to Yourself: Recognize that setbacks are natural. Don't be too harsh on yourself if you make a mistake. Instead, focused on your objectives and keep moving ahead.

Chapter 9
Exercise and Physical Activity

Complementing Your Diet with Fitness

Regular physical exercise, in addition to your Mayo Clinic Diet, is a great approach to improve your general health and expedite your weight loss and fitness objectives. Here are some ideas for adding exercise into your daily routine while adhering to the Mayo Clinic Diet:

1. Select an Exercise You like: Choose activities that you actually like. Walking, swimming, cycling, dancing, or participating in sports are all examples of pleasurable workouts that are more likely to become a regular part of your routine.
2. Begin Slowly: If you're new to fitness or haven't worked out in a while, start with low-intensity routines. As your fitness level increases, gradually increase the intensity and length.
3. Set Realistic Goals: Set attainable fitness goals that complement your diet and overall health objectives. Aim to exercise a set number of days each week, for example, or strive toward certain fitness goals.
4. Make a Schedule: Plan your workout sessions the same way you plan your meals. Having a routine makes it simpler to commit to exercises.

5. Combine Cardio and Strength Training: A well-rounded fitness regimen includes aerobic workouts (such as walking, running, or swimming) as well as strength training (such as weightlifting or bodyweight exercises). Cardiovascular exercise burns calories, but strength training develops muscle and increases metabolism.

6. Find a Workout Partner: Working out with a friend or family member may make exercise more enjoyable and give mutual encouragement and responsibility.

7. Make Use of Technology: Use fitness apps, monitors, or wearable gadgets to measure your progress and remain motivated. Many applications may assist you in setting and tracking fitness goals.

8. Participate in Fitness Classes or Groups: Attend group fitness classes or join a sports club or fitness community. The social side of exercise may make it more fun and help you remain consistent.

9. Establish It as a Habit: Consistency is essential. Incorporate exercise into your daily or weekly routine to make it a habit. Find a time that works best for you, whether it's in the morning, during lunch, or at night.

10. Track Your Progress: Track your exercise accomplishments in the same way you track your nutrition. Celebrate accomplishments

such as running a certain distance, lifting a greater weight, or increasing your endurance.

11. Rest and Recovery: Give your body time to recuperate between exercises. Rest is essential for avoiding injury and maintaining a steady habit.

12. Be Aware of Your Energy Balance: Consider the balance of calories ingested vs calories burnt during activity. Weight control is most successful when a nutritious diet is combined with frequent physical exercise.

Conclusion

In the last chapter of "The Mayo Clinic Diet Blueprint: Your Weight Loss Journey," it's time to reflect on your transforming journey and the useful lessons you've received. Inspired by the principles of the famous Mayo Clinic Diet, this book has given you with a thorough path to reach your weight reduction and general health objectives. In the last remarks, we recap the important insights and provide some final inspiration and encouragement.

Empowerment and Knowledge: Throughout this book, you've gained information and awareness of how to make educated, healthy food and lifestyle choices. You are no longer dependent on fad diets or quick remedies. You now have the insight to make long-term, sustainable adjustments.

Lifestyle Transformation: Your weight loss journey is about more than simply losing weight; it's about changing your whole way of life. It's about developing healthy eating habits, getting more exercise, and cultivating a good connection with food and your body.

Persistence and Commitment: We've stressed the need of constancy in your efforts. Your route to success will be to adhere to the principles of the Mayo Clinic Diet and to maintain a schedule of balanced eating and frequent exercise. The foundation of a healthy you is consistency.

Success Celebration: Take a minute to recognize your accomplishments, large and little. Every stride you've taken, every good decision you've made, and every challenge you've conquered deserves to be acknowledged. These accomplishments form the foundation for a better, happier future.

Above and Beyond the Scale: Your weight reduction journey is more than just the numbers on the scale. It is about greater vitality, self-esteem, mental and emotional well-being, and a lower chance of chronic illnesses. Accept the overall advantages of a healthy lifestyle.

Consistent Commitment: The Mayo Clinic Diet Blueprint has given you the tools, information, and direction you need. However, it is critical to recognize that your path is continuous. Continue to make good decisions, create and accomplish new objectives, and keep the healthy habits you've developed.

The Support System: On this journey, you are not alone. Lean on the encouragement of friends, family, and healthcare experts. Share your accomplishments, difficulties, and goals with others who care about your well-being.

A Better, Healthier Future: As you finish this book, imagine a future full with vivid health, vigor, and a lasting feeling of well-being. You have the blueprint for a healthy you, as well as the ability to design the life you want.

Remember, as you near the end of "The Mayo Clinic Diet Blueprint: Your Weight Loss Journey," that your journey is unique, and your route may vary from others. What counts most is your dedication to your health and your desire to live a meaningful life. The Mayo Clinic Diet laid the groundwork; now it's up to you to create the masterpiece that is your healthier, happier, and more vibrant future. Your adventure continues, and the options are endless. Accept it with open arms and a hopeful heart.